Intermittent Fasting for Women

The Essential Beginners Guide for Quick, Easy and Permanent Fat Loss

The information in the following pages is broadly considered to be a truthful and accurate account of facts and as such any inattention, use or misuse of the information in question by the reader will render any resulting actions solely under their purview. There are no scenarios in which the publisher or the original author of this work can be in any fashion deemed liable for any hardship or damages that may befall them after undertaking information described herein.

Additionally, the information in the following pages is intended only for informational purposes and should thus be thought of as universal. As befitting its nature, it is presented without assurance regarding its prolonged validity or interim quality. Trademarks that are mentioned are done without written consent and can in no way be considered an endorsement from the trademark holder.

Table of Contents

Introduction

There are so many strategies for losing weight. How do you know where to start? Women have different needs than men when it comes to dieting, exercise, and weight loss, and it seems that many popular strategies are aimed at men who want to look like muscular body builders. Many of these programs leave you hungry, unsatisfied, and ultimately lead to quitting early without ever seeing results.

Intermittent fasting is a natural way to make you feel and look better. Your body was designed to eat in this way and has been confused by the never-ending availability of food and snacks. This form of patterned eating will restore your energy levels, retain your needed body muscle while reducing body fat, and improve your overall health and wellness. The major problem with traditional diets is that they are just hard to stick to. You deny yourself your favorite food and snacks in hopes of weight loss and when you slip up, you feel ashamed and guilty—resulting in the derailment of your entire routine.

Cycling your eating pattern through periods of eating and fasting is as natural to your body as breathing. Humans have been eating this way for thousands of years, and only recently have we muddled our hunger signals so significantly that they are working against us instead of for us. Allowing yourself unrestricted access to food and snacks day in and day out alters your body's chemistry, increasing the production of hunger-signaling hormones. These hormones now tell your body constantly that you are hungry, and they are hard to ignore! Intermittent fasting will reprogram these hormones, decreasing your hunger signals and resigning them to the proper times of day.

Changing the way you eat is also difficult. By denying yourself your favorite meals, you are setting yourself up for failure. Intermittent fasting allows you to enjoy your favorite foods, snacks, and drinks as long as you are consuming them within your non-fasting window of time. Limiting the time you have available to consume calories will limit the total number of calories you'll ultimately consume—providing weight loss with little effort. Fasting for weight loss is different than a religious fast or fasting before a medical procedure. It does not mean you don't eat anything and wait for the pounds to fall off. You simply limit your total caloric intake during specific periods of time (hours of the day or days of the week, depending on which method if intermittent fasting you feel is most appropriate for you) while enjoying a normal diet and lifestyle the rest of the time! Reducing the amount of food you eat for short periods of time is simpler and easier to stick to for most women, resulting in success and dedication—without throwing in the towel.

The longer you practice intermittent fasting cycles, the easier you'll find them to be. Your body will adjust, you'll feel more motivation and energy, and you'll wonder how you could have possibly eaten the quantity of food you used to—all day long! This guide will explain in simple terms the science behind intermittent fasting, the benefits you can expect, and how to implement the plan into your life.

Chapter 1: Intermittent Fasting: Understanding the Basics

First things first. I've promised you success in your weight loss journey without calorie counting, traditional dieting, and hours upon hours of exercise. You aren't a muscular, bulky body builder—and you don't want to look like one! So, what am I asking you to do? Let's start with an overview of the basics, and then, we'll explore the method in greater detail throughout each chapter.

What is intermittent fasting?

Intermittent fasting is a pattern of providing your body the nutritional fuel it needs at specific time intervals each day. You will cycle through periods of alternately eating and fasting. Most of us do this in our daily lives anyway; we are simply extending these fasting periods between meals to reap the biggest weight loss and health benefits.

What is intermittent fasting NOT?

This practice of cycling your consumption is not a traditional diet. You will not be counting calories, eating the same thing every day, or being forced to spend hours doing complicated exercises. Intermittent fasting is not complicated or expensive, and it will not leave you feeling tired or sluggish.

Why practice intermittent fasting?

Fasting is generally regarded as a "four-letter word" (I know what you're thinking; "It actually has seven letters." Bear with me here.). We are about to change your entire mindset and understanding of weight loss, eating habits, and dieting. Throughout history, humans experienced fasting. At times, fasting was a way of life simply because food was not always available the way it is now. We can observe that both animals and humans will instinctively fast during times of great stress or illness. In certain regions of the world, religious groups mandate the practice of fasting as part of Islamic, Buddhist, and Christian customs. Practicing an intermittent fasting cycle is more natural to your biology than the typical three to four meals (and sometimes even more!) per day most of us are accustomed to. Your body is capable and even programmed to withstand extended instances of intense caloric restriction.

What are the benefits of intermittent fasting?

Multiple studies have shown that this pattern of eating can (and does!) produce weight loss, results in a marked improvement in metabolic health, promotes a longer life span, and aids in protecting the body against disease.

Let's review the basics of intermittent fasting in more detail.

Fasting is not, by any means, a new concept. We see fasting present in human history as well as in the natural world. Sometimes fasting was not a choice or instinct, but simply an occurrence throughout the lifetime of a human or animal. Times of drought or other impact would lead to a decrease in the availability of food at the lowest level of the food chain, and this scarcity would resonate throughout each subsequent level. In other instances of fasting, instinct or choice drives the desire to refrain from eating. When an animal or human suffers an illness, we can observe that fasting is an instinctual practice designed to help the body systems more readily fight disease.

There are written accounts as early as the period of 200 AD of fasting being recommended to treat illness. An important Greek philosopher, Plotinus, is reported to have suggested to a member of the Roman senate to only eat every other day to treat his gout. It is recorded that his patient's health increased, and eventually, the patient was cured of his affliction. While this is most likely not the first use of fasting as a medical treatment, it is one of the earliest written accounts we are able to consider today.

This understanding that fasting is and has been common throughout history serves to prove that this style of eating is certainly not a new phenomenon or fad, but should instead be seen as the rediscovery of a well-known concept.

So, when we speak of intermittent fasting the concept is based on a practice that has been around for thousands of years—the act of fasting. In our instance, you are intentionally avoiding food (and in some cases drinks—we'll get there later) for a set period of time. This intentionality and time frame are what separates a beneficial health practice like intermittent fasting from a negative unhealthy experience like starving.

Now that we know where the basis for the intermittent fasting concept originated, let's look at some evidence-based benefits it will provide to your health. There have been many scientific studies researching the effects of fasting on general health and wellness that have overwhelmingly produced positive conclusions.

Effects on cells, genes, and hormones

There are several things that occur within your body when you don't eat. To start, your body increases or decreases the production of certain hormones in order to make the stores of body fat more readily accessible. These are as follows:

- The levels of *insulin* circulating throughout your blood markedly decrease during fasting. This drop promotes the burning of fat stores in the body.[1]

- Blood levels of *human growth hormone* can rise as much as five times their normal levels during fasting. An increase in human growth hormone is linked to efficiency in fat utilization, muscle gain, among other benefits.[2]

- A period of fasting facilitates a *cellular repair* process vital to the body's continued health by removing waste products found within cells.[3]

- Fasting induces changes in gene expression within the body that relate to the healthy and successful aging of the brain[4] and protection from diseases, including certain types of cancer.[5]

Intermittent fasting is beneficial for weight loss and body composition.

For most women, practicing intermittent fasting will mean you eat fewer meals. As long as you are not overeating during the meals you do have, you'll generally end up consuming fewer calories than you are currently used to.

Add to this decrease in total calorie input the information we have already covered regarding the changes in insulin and hormones levels in the body, and you can see how this style of eating can enhance the body's ability to lose excess fat. When insulin levels are reduced and production of human growth hormone is increased, the body is more easily able to convert stored fat into usable energy, providing a 14% increase in your resting metabolic rate.[6] This increase in the body's metabolic process means that 14% more calories are being burned while you do nothing but rest. So, by following an eating pattern based on the concept of intermittent fasting you're attacking your problem of excess stored weight from two angles: not only is your body expending more energy during its daily processes due to the increase in metabolic rate, but you're also simply eating fewer calories. In 2012, a group of scientists reviewed the findings of multiple studies that were originally done to evaluate dietary methods for preventing diabetes. After looking at the results, they concluded that intermittent fasting alone can produce weight loss in the range of 3% to 8% over a period of 3–24 weeks.[7] The men and women in these studies also reportedly shrank their waist measurements by 4%–7%, indicating that they lost abdominal fat—a well-known predictor for disease.

Women generally tend to associate shedding pounds on the scale with slimming down and ultimately looking better. Most of you are not interested in building muscle mass like a weight lifter or body builder and would prefer to simply find a lifestyle eating plan that can help you reach your goals of looking better and feeling better. While you may not be interested in adding to your muscle mass, you do want to preserve the muscle you currently have in your body (everyone has some!). A downfall to traditional dieting methods you may have tried in the past is that continuous and extended calorie restriction usually results in a loss of body fat as well as muscle. In a study done in 2011 by the International Association for the Study of Obesity, researchers found that participants lost a relatively equal amount of weight on intermittent fasting programs and continuous calorie restriction programs, but those who followed an intermittent fasting cycle lost a smaller amount of muscle mass by the end.[8] Those who followed a traditional diet program where calorie consumption was limited over a long period of time showed 25% of their total weight loss to be muscle mass, whereas the individuals who followed an intermittent fasting cycle had only 10%.[8]

The important message to take away from all of this scientifically backed information is to understand that intermittent fasting is beneficial to your body on a cellular and genetic level, as well as physically. It will get you to your weight loss goal without restricting your calorie intake so much that you lose necessary muscle mass.

Intermittent fasting can lower your risk of type-2 diabetes.

There are more than 11 million women in the United States who have been diagnosed with diabetes.[9] Women generally fare worse than men when it comes to the long-term damage and side effects that diabetes causes to the body. If you are a woman diagnosed with diabetes, you are more likely to develop coronary heart disease, have a poorer quality of life, and have lower survival rates than men with the same condition. There is a clear connection between being overweight and the development of type-2 diabetes, and almost half (47%) of all women with diabetes have a body mass index greater than 30kg/m^2—officially classifying them as morbidly obese.[9]

Lowering blood sugar levels and keeping your body from becoming insulin resistant will help protect you from type-2 diabetes. Intermittent fasting can reduce blood sugar levels and benefit some women with an insulin resistance.[7] Studies done on humans show that during intermittent fasting cycles, blood sugar can be lowered by 3%–6% and insulin can be reduced by 20%–31%.[7] As is the case with any lifestyle change, every woman's body will react differently to fasting, so if you have already been diagnosed as diabetic or pre-diabetic it's important to discuss these changes with your doctor before you begin.

Intermittent fasting may benefit cardiovascular health.

Heart disease is currently at the top of the list as the leading cause of death in the United States for men and women.[10] There are risk factors specific to women that place you at a greater risk for developing heart disease. These include diabetes, stress, depression, smoking, inactivity, menopause, "broken heart syndrome", inactivity, and pregnancy.[10] General factors that place both men and women at higher risk include elevated cholesterol, elevated blood pressure, and obesity.[10] Intermittent fasting and the impact it can have on body systems have been studied in both human and animal subjects, and some of the research has shown it to have a beneficial effect on some of these heart disease risk factors. For example, lowering your risk of developing type-2 diabetes can also reduce your risk of developing heart disease as a result of diabetes complications. It has also been studied as a weight loss strategy in order to reduce the risk of developing coronary artery disease.[11]

Intermittent fasting can jumpstart repair processes within your cells.
Autophagy is the scientific term for the process of eliminating and recycling waste products from within cells. When you fast, specifically for short periods of time, this process is initiated and the cells within your body begin to get rid of dysfunctional components and waste that have built up within their walls.[12] There is some evidence showing that increasing this waste removal and recycling process may help protect you against Alzheimer's disease.[13]

Intermittent fasting may help reduce your risk of developing cancer.
Fasting may reduce your risk of developing certain types of cancer due to the beneficial effects it can have on the metabolism. More studies need to be done in this area of research, but so far, multiple animal-based studies have shown promising results related to short-term fasting and the prevention and treatment of certain cancers.[14,15]

You've now earned a basic understanding of idea surrounding the intermittent fasting concept including scientific evidence as to how it works, why it works, and how it may benefit you. The final step to completing your basic knowledge of the practice is to understand how to do it.

Methods of intermittent fasting

Over the years that intermittent fasting has been practiced by thousands of men and women, several methods have been created. Each of these various ways of following an intermittent fasting cycle produces the same overall outcome—to cycle your calorie consumption through periods of eating and fasting to lose weight and experience other health benefits associated with intermittent fasting. Finding the right method to work with your lifestyle will greatly increase your chance of success with intermittent fasting. Each of these methods will work better for some women than others, based on your daily schedule and preferred eating patterns.

Let's look at four popular methods of intermittent fasting.

1. **The 16/8 method:** This method is also known as the Leangains Protocol. To practice this style of intermittent fasting

you will skip breakfast and only consume your calories during an 8-hour period each day. For example, you will wake up in the morning and not eat breakfast. At 1:00 p.m., you may begin your calorie intake, and by 9:00 p.m., you will fast overnight (16 hours) until you begin the cycle again the next day. You may alter the hours of eating and fasting periods, but many women find it preferable to skip breakfast in the first part of their day and eat during the afternoon and evening hours. Finding a routine that works for you will be helpful in sticking with the intermittent fasting program.

Important points:

- You won't consume any calories during your fasting periods. It is acceptable to chew sugar-free gum, drink coffee with or without calorie-free sweeteners, and diet soda during this time, even though they may have a very small number of calories per serving.
- During your fasting period, you will experience an increase in energy. Use this time to get things done! Grocery shopping, housework, anything you have to do! Taking advantage of the energy boost by

being productive will motivate you to stick with the IF program and keep you from becoming preoccupied with food.

- The number of meals you have during your eating period does not matter. Most people will have three meals split up over these hours, but you can certainly have more or less. The fact that you are restricting your consumption of calories from all day to an 8-hour window should decrease the total number of calories you are able to consume daily.
- Your body will get used to eating during certain times of the day, so keeping consistent with your eating and fasting periods will help you to regulate your hunger to the appropriate times of day.
- This method is generally considered easy to follow because it can be as simple as not snacking after you've finished eating dinner and skipping breakfast the next morning before resuming your normal eating habits.
- It is frequently recommended that women shorten the fasting length to 14–15 hours if 16 hours is difficult to adhere to.

2. **The Eat/Stop/Eat method:** This method of intermittent fasting has you fast for an entire day (24 hours) two times per week.

   Important points:

   - For example: You would eat dinner, and then not eat again until dinner time the next night.
   - Breakfast to breakfast or lunch to lunch fasting will also produce the same result.
   - Coffee with zero-calorie sweeteners, water, zero-calorie sodas, and sugar-free gum are allowed during the fasting period.
   - This method may be difficult for some women to stick to. If you prefer this method, you may find it easier to start with a shorter fasting period (16 hours) and work up to the 24-hour period.

3. **The 5:2 method:** Following this method involves choosing days of the week (not back to back days) that you will consume between 500 and 600 calories for the entire day. The other days of the week you will eat normally.

Important points:

- As with most intermittent fasting cycle protocols, there are no specific requirements of *what* to eat but rather *when* to eat, but binging or overeating can hinder your weight loss.
- This method is simple because 5 days in a week, you will eat as you normally do. On your two non-consecutive fasting days, you will consume 1/4 of your normal calorie intake, roughly 500 calories per day for most women.
- An example would be to plan three small meals for Monday and Thursday each week (approximately 500 calories total) and then eat normally on Tuesdays, Wednesdays, Fridays, Saturdays, and Sundays.
- Eating "normally" on your non-fasting days should include an average diet. You don't want to binge on large amounts of junk foods those days or overeat.
- Water, coffee with zero-calorie sweetener, zero-calorie soda, and sugar-free gum may be consumed during the fasting period.

4. **The Warrior Diet:** This method was made popular by a well-known expert in the fitness world named Ori Hofmekler. In this method, you fast during the day and break your fast with a large meal at night.

   Important points:

   - You may eat a few fruits and vegetables during your daytime fasting period as long as they are uncooked, raw snacks.
   - You have a 4-hour window of time in the evening where you will eat. You may eat normally as many times as you would like during this 4-hour period, and the idea is to "feast" to prepare you for your fasting period the next day.
   - This method of intermittent fasting is usually paired with dietary choices that adhere to the paleo diet style of nutrition. Acceptable foods are mostly whole, unprocessed foods that are similar to their natural state.

5. **Spontaneously skipping meals:** This method is probably the simplest and easiest to follow. All you must do is skip

meals when you're just not hungry, or when it's convenient to do so.

Important points:

- This method is not structured like some of the others, but will still provide benefits of intermittent fasting.
- Skip meals occasionally, whenever you don't feel hungry or are too busy to cook anything.
- So, if you're not hungry when you wake up one morning, skip breakfast. Eat a healthy lunch and dinner. Or, if you're traveling and it's easier to skip lunch than to stop somewhere, just continue your travels and eat dinner when you have more time.
- Skipping a meal or two when it is convenient or when you just feel like it is a spontaneous fast can reinvigorate your metabolism and provide the same benefits of fasting that a planned fast can.

There has been some evidence that when women fast, the production of certain hormones is increased in response to a woman's sensitivity to hunger signals. So, as a woman tries to fast, her body ramps up production of the hormones that produce hunger signals, making her even more hungry! If you find these methods not quite working for you, you may benefit from trying a combination of these intermittent fasting protocols known as crescendo fasting for women. This method is like the above methods, but you will fast on two or three non-consecutive days (e.g., Tuesday, Thursday, and Saturday.) for 12–16 hours per day.

Consider your own lifestyle and eating preferences. Remember that unlike traditional diets, intermittent fasting is less dependent on what foods you eat and relies more heavily on what time and how often you eat. You may want to test out a few different methods before deciding which cycle works best for you. Finding a protocol that will work in between your busy schedule and be compatible with your body's rhythm is critically important to the success of reaching your goals through the use of intermittent fasting.

Chapter 2: Dietary and Exercise Considerations for Intermittent Fasting

How will your diet affect your weight loss goals while practicing intermittent fasting?
In the previous chapter, we covered the basics of intermittent fasting, and by now, you should understand that the main concept of following an intermittent fasting cycle has more to do with when you consume calories and less to do with where those calories are coming from.

The weight loss benefit of practicing this kind of cycled eating comes from not only stimulating your metabolism and other bodily processes through fasting but simply from having less time to consume as many calories as you would during a normal day. Most people tend to snack throughout the day, eat at least three large meals, and may even consume calories at night through snacks or drinks. By putting a limit on the length of time that calories are to be taken in, most people will drastically reduce the total number of calories per day. Grazing is a term used to describe the pattern of eating that many women find themselves doing, whether they know it or not. Unrestricted access to food is common in today's culture and is putting you at great risk for over consumption of calories—leading to continued weight gain. If you're someone who is used to this style of constant snacking and unrestricted eating, your body has grown accustomed to being fed all day long. This leads to a continual sensation of hunger and the urge to eat at all times throughout the day, rather than just at meal times. It can take some time to retrain your body and brain to limit hunger signals to the appropriate times of day. Sticking to your intermittent fasting eating pattern will continue to feel easier each time you complete a fasting cycle.

If you have a normal diet, meaning you eat an average amount of food and don't partake in routinely binge or overeating, you should notice weight loss benefits from intermittent fasting without making changes to the foods you eat. This is one of the greatest perks of following the intermittent fasting "diet"! For many women, a diet has traditionally involved restricting calories for an extended period of time. Not only is this method of weight loss difficult to stick to—limiting the percentage of those who comply long term—but when you extendedly restrict calories, you create a reliance on high-quality nutrition as well. This is a major hang-up for many people who don't have the time to consistently prepare varied and nutritionally dense meals multiple times per day, as well as for those who are just unfamiliar with nutritional science and nutrient needs. Counting calories doesn't take into account the interactions within the body that are specific to every person and their diet. It can lead to a preoccupation with tracking foods consumed versus calories spent, creating mental stress and anguish—a contributing factor to the stalling of weight loss!

By following an intermittent fasting protocol, you don't have to worry about tracking how many calories you consume and logging your exercise to determine how many you've expended. You don't have to swear off your favorite snack foods, and you don't have to restrict yourself to only consuming nutritionally dense foods that you don't have to prepare or that you just don't like. Following your normal diet but planning it around specific hours will jumpstart your metabolism and ultimately provide the weight loss you've been looking for. Intermittent fasting cycling simplifies dieting and weight loss so that *everyone* and *anyone* can lose weight! You don't have to worry about preparing and cooking ealth foods, purchasing overpriced s or meal replacements, or spending ...ssing over certain foods and denying yourself your favorite snacks and treats.

If you find that during your periods of eating you tend to take in a large amount of junk food or you tend to overcompensate for your periods of fasting, you may want to consider making a few dietary changes to help you lose more weight quickly. While intermittent fasting simplifies dieting by eliminating the need to count calories and follow a strict dieting plan, consuming far too many calories will not provide weight loss. It is a simplified, effective weight loss tool, but it is not a magic solution to eating anything and everything you want in great quantity and lose weight! There is no magic solution, and if a diet program ever promises to be one, you should run the other way as fast as you can! It is a generally understood concept that too many calories in and not enough calories expended will not lead to weight loss, and depending on the difference between the two can even lead to weight gain. Even with the increase in resting metabolic function from the act of fasting intermittently won't completely negate an abnormally high-calorie diet during the non-fasting hours. When you first begin your intermittent fasting cycle, it may be helpful to keep an eye on the kinds of foods you're consuming during your "normal" days and your non-fasting periods, as well as the quantity. If you feel you may be overeating during these times or choosing mainly high-calorie foods, you can consider making a few dietary changes in order to fully benefit from the effects of your intermittent fasting cycles.

While not required, you may choose to make changes to your diet in order to experience the most benefits from intermittent fasting in the shortest amount of time. There are no specific nutritional requirements that the intermittent fasting protocol relies on, but a general focus on foods that are less processed can increase the quality of your calories and result in faster and speedier weight loss.

Does exercise play a role in intermittent fasting?

As promised, intermittent fasting will produce weight loss for most women regardless of the incorporation of an exercise regimen. Pairing your intermittent fasting cycle with a lifestyle that isn't sedentary will be enough. Not sitting for long periods of time and regular movement are both important factors in any healthy lifestyle and any diet routine aimed at weight loss.

Regular movement and even exercise can be an important aspect of any weight loss plan, but exercise alone won't cancel out continuously poor dietary choices. The foods you consume have a greater impact on regulation of weight than does your physical activity or fitness.

So, the bottom line is that most women don't *need* to exercise to lose weight while practicing intermittent fasting, but if you *want* to incorporate structured exercise into your routine, there are certain activities that can give you the most "bang for your buck". Plus, as an added bonus, exercise can be a temporary appetite suppressor, and one study of overweight participants showed that those who engaged in physical activity every other day while following an intermittent fasting program lost more weight than the group that didn't.

The best exercise routine to pair with your intermittent fasting cycle is to visit the gym three times per week and perform a brief warm up, a weightlifting routine, and a few cool down and stretching poses. Now, I know what you're thinking. Don't be intimidated by the mention of exercise or weightlifting. As promised, the addition of regimented physical activity to your cycled eating is optional, and you may find you don't need or wish to incorporate it into your intermittent fasting practices. The beauty of this plan is in its universal effectiveness—it can benefit *everyone* from *body builders* to *you*!

For those who are interested in a workout routine that will optimize their weight loss while following an intermittent fasting eating plan, I've simplified the science behind these specific exercises as well as created an easy-to-follow regimen that will provide you with confidence at the gym. And of course, you don't need to worry about these weightlifting exercises making you appear bulky or muscular, they are specifically geared toward women's bodies and, when combined with intermittent fasting, can help you achieve a toned, healthy look!
Lifting weights will burn calories while providing an extra boost to your metabolism (on top of the increased metabolic stimulation intermittent fasting provides.). Studies have shown that even while actively following a diet plan and losing weight, weightlifting can build muscle.[16]

Simplified exercise plan for women

Rules for incorporating simple exercise into your intermittent fasting weight loss routine:

- On the days you are fasting, do light physical activity like yoga, low-intensity swimming, or light cardio like a brisk walk or slow jog.
- On the days you are not fasting, do more intense physical activity like high-intensity interval training or weight lifting.
- Drink plenty of water when doing physical activity, on fasting and non-fasting days!

An example of a high-intensity interval training exercise can be as simple as follows:

Three rounds: 20 seconds of exercise and 10 seconds of rest between each exercise.

1. Air boxing: Stand with your right foot slightly in front of your left and your hips pointed toward your left side. Set your arms in a boxer's stance and punch with your right arm toward your left side, and then punch with your left arm headed toward your right side. Repeat.
2. Air boxing (again): Rotate your stance so that your left foot is slightly in front of your right and your hips point toward your right side. Again, take your boxer's stance and punch with your left arm first followed by your right.
3. Jumping jacks: Simply do as many jumping jacks as you can do in the 20 seconds of allotted time.
4. Squats: Do as many squats as you can in the 20 seconds of allotted time, ensuring you are squatting deep enough to feel your thigh muscles begin to tire.

An example of a simple weight training routine for women:

A weight lifting routine for women does not have to be complicated, heavy, or produce bulky results. Engaging your muscles in weight lifting activity will keep your bones strong and healthy, lower your risks of osteoarthritis, and build muscle mass, thus increasing the speed of your metabolism and providing you with the toned arms and legs that most women seek. Weight lifting does not always have to include lifting actual weights! Bodyweight exercises are incredibly effective for slightly increasing a woman's muscle mass and shaping her body.

Always warm up before beginning your routine!

Start by doing squats. Try doing somewhere between 8 and 12 squats, take a small rest, and repeat one more time.

Use one light dumbbell in each hand (approximately 8 pounds) to do two sets of rows, somewhere between 8 and 12 rows per set. Stand with your feet apart, in line with your knees, and your knees slightly bent. Keep your back flat and lean forward from your hips. Lift the weights up to your chest while pulling your shoulders back. Your elbows should be bent and pointed backward while your palms face in.

Next, use your body weight to do push-ups. Start out doing them on your knees, and move to a full push-up whenever you feel capable. Again, do two sets of 8 to 12 push-ups, increasing the number as you gain strength and are able.

Finally, end your routine with a plank. To do this, you'll hold your chest off the floor with your forearms, while your toes face the floor. Lower your waist toward the floor until your body becomes a straight line, parallel to the floor. Start by holding this position for as long as you can, eventually working your way up to a 60-second hold.

Don't be intimidated by the incorporation of exercise into your intermittent fasting routine. Increasing your physical activity will benefit your weight loss and provide an even greater boost of energy. Don't feel that you need to start everything at once! You may find it easier to begin your fasting routine for a few weeks before you add in an exercise routine. The most important aspect of any weight loss program is to do what works for you! This will increase the likelihood that you'll stick with it long enough to see results.

Chapter 3: Intermittent Fasting and Social Situations

Let's address the social aspect of your new eating plan and healthy lifestyle. Often, many women can be rude and even cruel when dieting, losing weight, and making healthy lifestyle changes becomes a topic of conversation. Most people are not familiar with the body's nutritional needs or with the benefits that intermittently fasting can provide. They don't understand the body's capacity to benefit from these periods of restricted eating, and they certainly can't understand why skipping breakfast would ever be part of a healthy weight loss regimen! Most people have been trained their entire lives to falsely believe that breakfast is the most important meal of the day. When they hear you're purposely skipping breakfast, they can even act maliciously toward you and put you down, no matter how much (or really, how little!) they know about diet, exercise, and how the body functions.

So, you've got a few options when it comes to how to respond in social situations to comments or attitudes regarding your intermittent fasting cycles. Being prepared can help you to feel more comfortable and confident should questions or comments arise among friends or family while you are in your non-eating period of your fasting cycle.

First, and possibly most obvious, is to decide if you will attend a certain social function or situation during your fasting period. If you feel more comfortable skipping an event to avoid questions or unfavorable attitudes in response to your cycled eating, it may be a more favorable option for you.

However, sometimes you may be unable to refrain from attending an event, or maybe you'll eventually be subject to questioning from family members or coworkers in the lunch room. So, how should you respond to social interactions and situations as someone who practices intermittent fasting?

Don't tell them you're fasting.

The simplest solution to avoid negative comments, intrusive questions, and unwanted "advice" is to avoid telling people about your fasting. This solution is relatively easy and keeps the subject from coming up or opening yourself up to criticism. Especially when others hear that you've skipped breakfast, negative comments and judgments tend to follow.

If the subject does come into conversation, perhaps your significant other or friend mentions to someone else that you skipped breakfast that day, an easy and effective option is to simply use an excuse.

Your excuses:

- "I've just never been very hungry for breakfast in the morning."
  This is an acceptable excuse for a surprisingly large amount of people. Most people just ignore their own hunger signals (or lack of) because they've been groomed to believe breakfast is "the most important meal of the day", but almost everyone has had the experience of just not being hungry for a meal.
- "I'm doing a detox."
  This is also a highly accepted answer to questions regarding your lack of food consumption in a social setting. Detoxing has become mainstream in recent years thanks to celebrities and the media. Most people have heard that detoxing is beneficial to your body, and whether they themselves agree with the practice or not,

they understand that it is socially acceptable to wish to remove toxins from the body by way of a detox. Intermittent fasting is a great way to start the process of waste removal from body cells, so this "excuse" is factually based and a good option.

How to respond in specific social situations

If someone invites you to meet them for breakfast, just go! Don't let your new eating pattern and the fact that you are improving your health by foregoing breakfast that day keep you from enjoying the company of your family and friends. Go out to breakfast, order water with lemons, tea, or coffee.

If someone asks you why you aren't ordering food, simply use one of the excuses listed above. It's rather rare that someone will continue to press you about your dietary choices, but on occasion, it is bound to happen. In this case and you happen to be in the company of someone who won't stop questioning your decision to not order, it's perfectly polite and acceptable to respond with something like "I'm very happy with my coffee and catching up with you. It's more important to me to spend time with you than it is to order breakfast." Most people will stop questioning you after saying something like this.

Situations you might find yourself in that kind of questioning are social events involving bars or alcohol. If you happen to be invited to an event on one of your fasting days, you don't have to worry about declining the invitation. If you worry that someone may comment on your drinking (or lack of) there are some techniques you can use to deflect the unwanted questioning and attention. If you're at a loud or crowded bar, it should be easy to get a glass of water with a lime. Anyone seeing you with your drink will assume it's a gin and tonic, and no one will even make a comment! If you're at a table with friends you can still order the same thing, but be prepared to be asked why you aren't drinking. Just tell them you don't feel like drinking, your stomach hurts, or any number of excuses you can come up with on the spot. Most friends won't push you for further information and will quickly move on to the next topic of conversation.

When you're currently in a fasting period you'll want to be prepared with your excuses or your answers to the questions you're sure to get from friends and family about your lack of eating or ordering food. So, let's do a simple recap of your go-to solutions for dealing with this problem:

1. Don't tell people you're fasting!

2. If the secret spills, tell them you're just not hungry or you're doing a detox.
3. If someone insists you order food, complement them on their company and conversation and order a water, tea, or coffee.
4. If your plans include alcohol or a bar, use the mock gin and tonic, or the excuse that you just don't feel like drinking. Everyone has felt this way at one point or another!

Finally, if all else fails and someone continues to press you about your eating patterns or your lack of eating during a certain time, the best choice is to be honest with them. Explain to them what you're doing and why you're doing it, and include scientifically based research and facts as to why it works for you. Don't allow negative comments and judgments from others to derail your progress or take your focus off your weight loss goals. You know what is best for you and your body, and you are fully capable of listening to it and caring for yourself properly.

Chapter 4: Specific Considerations When Implementing Intermittent Fasting

You've now got a thorough understanding of the background of intermittent fasting, the scientifically based evidence of its benefits, how to do it, and how to work this cycle of eating into your own life.

There are some considerations as to who may or may not benefit from intermittent fasting. There are a lot of women (and men) who have gotten great weight loss results using some form of fasting and cycled eating. However, just like any diet and exercise program or regimen, intermittent fasting is not for everyone, and it's important you practice the proper weight loss plan for your body and your specific goals. Intermittent fasting is certainly not something that everyone needs to do, but it's a helpful tool in the weight loss battle that so many women struggle with. It can be easily implemented in many women's daily lives and used to promote greater overall health and well-being, but it can, in some cases, be misused as well.

There are a few pre-requisites that if followed, will make your intermittent fasting weight loss journey *easier* and *more successful*, and make you a good candidate for reaping the *most* benefits from this program. These include the following:

- Get enough sleep on a regular basis.
- Minimize stress in your daily life.
- Make sure lifestyle activity is within a normal range—not too much or too little daily movement and/or exercise.
- Be fat adapted. This means that your body can easily access and burn stored fat throughout the day when it's needed to provide energy.

So, how can you tell if you're already considered fat adapted? There is no blood test that can give you this answer, but there are a few simple questions you can ask yourself that should be able to provide you with an indication of your level of fat adaptability:

- Can you go 3 hours or more without eating? Would skipping a meal be an incredibly difficult physical and mental struggle for you?

- On a normal day, do you feel your energy level stays consistent throughout the day? Do you need to take an afternoon nap or is it just something you enjoy doing now and again?

- Are you able to perform fairly vigorous physical activity like steady walking, jogging, or light exercise without first consuming carbohydrates for energy?

- Do you frequently suffer from headaches, mental exhaustion, and mental fog?

Someone whose body is fat adapted can usually skip meals with little effort on their part. They have consistent energy and do not require an afternoon nap to make it through the second portion of their day. They are able to be moderately active and perform physical activities like brisk walking, jogging, hiking, biking, and swimming without needing to fuel their body beforehand with carbohydrates, and they do not suffer from the mental fog, headaches, and exhaustion that a person whose body is more sugar dependent may.

Some of you are lucky and are genetically predisposed to be a fat burning machine! Others of you may not be, and your genetics may require more effort than the first group to reach this state of fat burning and freedom from sugar and carbohydrate dependence. Luckily for all of us, your genes are not final! They don't define you, and they can be altered! Through your behavior and your lifestyle choices, you have the ability to turn on and off various genes in your genetic code that can lead to the physical results you desire. There are numerous versions of the future person you may become, and it's always up to you to make the decisions that will ultimately lead to who you will become. You are responsible for making choices and living a lifestyle that will promote and direct your genes toward fat loss, building muscle, and overall wellness. Following an intermittent fasting style of eating will put you on the path to achieving this longevity of life and general wellness of the body.

If you feel that you may be lacking in the fat-adaptability department and want to give yourself the best start to your intermittent fasting protocol, it can benefit you to try eating the paleo style diet for 3 weeks before beginning your cycles of fasting and eating. This basically means you'll eliminate sugar, grains, legumes, and vegetable oils from your diet for 3 weeks prior to beginning intermittent fasting. This should be the push your body needs to become more efficient in drawing upon fat stores for energy rather than relying on dietary sugar for fuel. Again, this step is *not necessary* for your pursuit of weight loss through intermittent fasting, but it can set you up for the most success in the shortest amount of time.

Are there any indicators of someone whom intermittent fasting may not be beneficial for?

Intermittent fasting *may not* be a great protocol to follow for someone who is susceptible to eating disorders. If you've had a problem with disordered eating at any point in your life, it might be beneficial for you to explore multiple weight loss plans before deciding what works best for you. If intermittent fasting seems like the best choice for your lifestyle, do take the time to pay special attention to the amount of food you're consuming when you are not in your fasting periods, just to be sure you're not continuously denying yourself nutrition.

Intermittent fasting is considered a stressor on your body systems. You're using planned fasting and hunger to ignite metabolic processes within your body that respond to these stressors. For this reason, someone with a multitude of other stressors may not fare as well while following an intermittent fasting protocol. Mental stress, physical stress, and emotional stress can all hinder your mental ability to properly complete your fasting cycles as well as your body's physical ability to lose weight. Adding this new stressor can compound any other existing stressors, which won't be the most effective way to begin your weight loss journey.

Intermittent fasting may not be beneficial for someone with a cortisol regulation disorder. If you're actively monitoring your cortisol levels with your doctor or if you think you may have an issue with cortisol regulation it would be best to seek a professional opinion before implementing a fast into your weight loss regimen. Fasting raises cortisol levels in the body, and in a healthy individual, this poses no threat or health issue. Someone with a cortisol dysregulation can have serious side effects if their levels become excessive, and an activity that boosts production of cortisol may not be right for these people. If you think you may have an issue with cortisol regulation, visit your doctor before starting a program and find out for sure. You may have an issue with cortisol regulation if you retain excess belly fat, consistently lack enough sleep, persistently suffer from low-grade stress, and rely on caffeine to keep you awake and energized each day.

Should a pregnant woman practice intermittent fasting?

There haven't been many studies done on the effects of fasting by pregnant women on their growing fetus. One study[17] that followed pregnant women fasting for Ramadan showed that these women had a decrease in the development and growth of their placentas, but the slower growth was more efficient. The developing fetus grew as normal, but the women had much smaller reserves of nutrients in their bodies. Although this (and a few other) studies show that short-term fasting is probably safe during pregnancy, it is most likely a better idea to wait until after giving birth. Fasting during pregnancy is not necessary (except in these cases of religiously required fasts) and is probably not beneficial to the woman or her growing baby.

Should I fast if I am a diabetic?

This is a gray area and should be reviewed with your doctor before you begin. Women generally have a more difficult time regulating their blood sugar than men and can be more severely affected by a drop in blood sugar. There have been accounts of men who were classified as diabetic using intermittent fasting to control their blood sugar levels, lose weight, and effectively beat type-2 diabetes, but there have been no such accounts for women.

Will intermittent fasting affect my menstrual cycle and fertility?

Humans are highly biologically effective at adapting to their environments. When proper nutrition is not available, it is more work for a woman's body to create new life and provide nutrition for the baby once it's born. For this reason, women are biologically designed to respond to the presence or scarcity of available food by altering some aspects of fertility. There haven't been clinical studies directly comparing the effects of intermittent fasting on female fertility. These studies do have to look at, mostly, and compare fertility changes due to extreme fasting circumstances like famine or anorexia—which are not truly comparable to planned and purposeful intermittent fasting. These studies do show a link between decreased fertility, the loss of a menstrual cycle, and fasting, but the differences between these scenarios and intermittent fasting should be considered. There is currently too little evidence-based clinical information on the relationship between intermittent fasting and female reproductive health to definitively say if it is beneficial, neutral, or harmful.

So, now you might be wondering—Is intermittent fasting right for me?

The short answer: It depends.

The long answer: As with any diet or exercise program, intermittent fasting is a lifestyle change. If you have medical conditions that are already present, it's best that you first check with your doctor if this style of eating is right for you. If you're pregnant, over stressed, struggling with insomnia, or have a history of an eating disorder intermittent fasting may not be the most appropriate weight loss solution for you.

If you're otherwise healthy and you're looking to lose weight and increase your general wellness, intermittent fasting can be a helpful tool in what seems like a never-ending battle.

Chapter 5: Myths About Intermittent Fasting

There are many myths being shared about intermittent fasting diets and their effectiveness or lack thereof. Looking at some of the more common ones floating around will not only help you in deciding if intermittent fasting is the right weight loss tool for you, but it will prepare you in case you may encounter them in social situations.

1. **Intermittent fasting will slow down your metabolism, making it harder for you to lose weight.**

   This myth that the frequency of eating your meals will slow down your metabolism and put your body into "starvation mode" is extremely common and well known. There is a ton of research supporting the claim that no matter how many times you're eating per day, if the calorie amount is consistent, your rate of metabolism will be unaffected.

2. **Intermittent fasting breaks down muscle in the body to use as energy.**

   Everyone needs some muscle in their body, even average women who have zero interest in looking like a body builder. Muscle development does impact your metabolic rate, gives you strength, and confidence, and is responsible for the body shape that most women wish to achieve. So, of course, we don't want to do anything that will encourage the body to draw upon muscle mass for energy. Studies have shown that as long as you are using your muscle mass (even in the form of light to moderate physical activity), your muscles will not break down and disappear even in the presence of an extended period of fasting.[18]

3. Skipping breakfast makes you gain weight.

Everyone has heard this one! You'll probably hear it a dozen more times while following your intermittent fasting lifestyle. There is a myth that has been around for many years that there is something special about breakfast. So, many men and women falsely believe that skipping breakfast will lead to weight gain. There have been studies done that observed the connection between people who regularly skip breakfast and their weight showing that there is, in fact, a *statistical* correlation between skipping this meal and being overweight or obese. This is probably explained by the fact that the average person skipping breakfast is less health conscious and nutrition-savvy in general. A study done in 2014[19] compared overweight and obese subjects who ate breakfast and those who didn't. After 16 weeks, there was no difference in the weight of either group.

4. **Intermittent fasting is bad for your overall health.**

Throughout this book, we've looked at numerous evidence-based examples of why this is simply not true. There are a variety of benefits provided to your body from planned and timed fasting including protection against cancer and Alzheimer's disease, weight loss, mental clarity, detoxification of cells within the body, simplification of a diet and nutritional routine, increased energy, and more!

5. **Intermittent fasting will make you overeat, causing you to gain weight.**

Some people claim that you won't lose weight using intermittent fasting because you'll overcompensate during your eating periods and eat more than you would normally. This can be true, and some people do tend to eat slightly more after breaking a fast than they would have normally eaten had they not been fasting. An analysis of people following a fasting protocol was studied and showed that those who fasted for an entire 24 hours ended up taking in about 500 extra calories the next day. So, these people expended (or used up) about 2,400 calories during their fasting day, and the next day, they "overcompensated" by consuming an "extra" 500 calories. So, taking all of this information into account, these people actually had a 1,900 calorie deficit over a 2-day period, which is a substantial deficit in a short period of time and would lead to significant weight loss. Other studies have shown that fasting for a period of 3–24 weeks (with no dietary changes or exercise included) can decrease belly fat anywhere from 4% to 7% and cause a weight loss of 0.55 lbs–1.65 lbs per week.[7]

6. Intermittent fasting is only for men and women who want to be bodybuilders.

This last myth couldn't be farther from the truth! Intermittent fasting is not a diet, and it's not specific to any one gender, type of person, or lifestyle. It's for any person who wants to simplify the complicated world of dieting and nutrition to lose weight and gain overall good health. It doesn't require heavy workouts, intense exercise, or hours of pre-planning meals. It can be easily incorporated into your daily life, whether you work full time or stay at home with your children. There are various methods of intermittent fasting, and the beauty of this weight loss program is that you are able to use the eating plan that works with your specific schedule and your specific dietary needs!

Chapter 6: Get Started Today!

You've got everything you need now to get started losing weight, feeling better, and getting healthier using intermittent fasting. All you have to do now is start!

Step 1: Evaluate your current health and your goals.
Start by looking at your overall health as it currently stands. If you have any special concerns (like diabetes or other medical and health issues), review your new intermittent fasting intentions with your doctor to be sure you're healthy enough to begin. Determine how much weight you want to lose and set a realistic completion date. Once you begin practicing intermittent fasting and monitoring the speed at which you drop pounds, you can alter your goal and your completion date or incorporate an exercise routine to speed up your weight loss.
Step 2: Identify which method of intermittent fasting will work best for your lifestyle and goals.
Read through the important information about each method of intermittent fasting. Consider your schedule, your lifestyle, and what you think might be easiest for you. You may consider trying

a few different methods before deciding on the one that will be most effective for you. Remember, with each method, you can customize the fasting and eating hours to fit your preferences and schedule. The time of day of your fasting and when you eat is not what's important, so plan to break your fasts on days and during hours that will be convenient and easiest for you to stick to.

Step 3: Start!

Once you've decided on a method you're ready to start. Keep a journal or a log of the times and days you plan to fast and when you'll be eating. This can help to keep you on track when you start, but won't be necessary for the long term. Your body will adjust to your new pattern of eating, and your hunger signals will soon be all the reminder you need that it's time to break your most recent fasting cycle!

Step 4: Monitor your weight loss and incorporate an exercise routine for faster results.

If you're perfectly happy with the amount of weight intermittent fasting provides you per week, you may decide not to add a daily exercise routine. Normal physical activity including daily walks may be enough for many women to lose weight while using intermittent fasting. If you feel your weight loss could use a push, refer to the chapter on exercise during intermittent fasting and create a physical activity schedule and routine that you'll stick to. Keep in mind that it usually takes your body about 2 weeks to adjust to this new cycle of eating and fasting. Until then, you may experience frequent hunger signals while your body regulates the hormones responsible for appetite—this is normal and expected. Your body chemistry has been altered by the constant availability of food and has responded with an overproduction of hunger-producing hormones. One of the goals of intermittent fasting is to reprogram these hormones and regulators back to their original state. This way, your body will send hunger signals when it's truly in need of nutrition—something, many women can't even remember experiencing!

It's as simple as that. As promised, intermittent fasting really is the weight loss strategy that can be adapted to anyone's lifestyle or goals. No special diet is required, and no lengthy exercise program is needed, but both can certainly be incorporated to boost your total weight loss.

Conclusion

You should now understand how intermittent fasting can be beneficial to your weight loss goals. It's one of the most popular trends in the health and fitness world today, frequently being used by all different women to lose weight, simplify their lives, and improve their health. The best way to get started is to follow the steps within this guide to start today. Evaluate your goals and your needs and contemplate the best way to incorporate intermittent fasting into your lifestyle. Once you begin you'll see that your worries and fears will quickly disintegrate, just like your extra body fat! This method of losing weight really is for anyone, including you! Don't let your mental excuses and hang-ups keep you from achieving the body you want and the good health you deserve.

Remember: *intermittent fasting is not a diet!* It's simply a pattern of eating and fasting to retrain your body to run efficiently–the way it was designed to. This style of eating works and has been proven time and time again through various studies and research. It simplifies your life, reducing your three plus meals per day (plus snacks in between) to a smaller, more manageable amount, requiring less time in the kitchen wondering what "diet" foods to prepare today.

The psychological component of intermittent fasting will enable you to become more aware of what a real hunger signal is. Many women don't truly know the difference between their body signaling that it is time to refuel and their mind being accustomed to eating or snacking. This is one of the biggest challenges and largest hurdles to overcome for most women at the beginning of their intermittent fasting journey. Acknowledging that this is an issue that will need to be understood and addressed will help you overcome any intrusive thoughts about throwing in the towel too soon.

While this comprehensive guide to intermittent fasting is certainly detailed, there are so many aspects of health, wellness, dieting, and fitness that are complementary to this style of eating. Continue your weight loss journey by pursuing a greater understanding of these supplemental facets of wellness. Experiment with new recipes and new exercises that can increase your weight loss and add years and quality to your life.

Take control of your health and wellness using intermittent fasting like so many others have. The hardest part of any lifestyle change is just to get started. Once you begin to see results, you'll be motivated to stick with it, and soon, you'll be experiencing the weight loss and health benefits you've always dreamed of!

End Notes

Heilbronn, L. K., S. R. Smith, C. K. Martin, S. D. Anton, and E. Ravussin. Alternate-day fasting in nonobese subjects: Effects on body weight, body composition, and energy metabolism. *The American Journal of Clinical Nutrition*. January 2005. Accessed April 14, 2017.
https://www.ncbi.nlm.nih.gov/pubmed/15640462.

[2] **Ho, K. Y., J. D. Veldhuis, M. L. Johnson, R. Furlanetto, W. S. Evans, K. G. Alberti, and M. O. Thorner. Fasting enhances growth hormone secretion and amplifies the complex rhythms of growth hormone secretion in man. *Journal of Clinical Investigation*. April 1988. Accessed April 14, 2017. https://www.ncbi.nlm.nih.gov/pmc/articles/PMC329619/.**

[3] **Alirezaei, Mehrdad, Christopher C. Kemball, Claudia T. Flynn, Malcolm R. Wood, J. Lindsay Whitton, and William B. Kiosses. Short-term fasting induces profound neuronal autophagy. *Autophagy*. August 16, 2010. Accessed April 14, 2017.**
https://www.ncbi.nlm.nih.gov/pmc/articles/PMC3106288/.

[4] **Martin, Bronwen, Mark P. Mattson, and Stuart Maudsley. Caloric restriction and intermittent fasting: Two potential diets for successful brain aging. *Ageing Research Reviews*. August 2006. Accessed April 14, 2017. https://www.ncbi.nlm.nih.gov/pmc/articles/PMC2622429/.**

[5] **Zhu, Y., Y. Yan, D. R. Gius, and A. Vassilopoulos. Metabolic regulation of Sirtuins upon fasting and the implication for cancer. *Current Opinion in Oncology*. November 2013. Accessed April 14, 2017.** https://www.ncbi.nlm.nih.gov/pubmed/24048020.

[6] **Mansell, P. I., I. W. Fellows, and I. A. Macdonald. Enhanced thermogenic response to epinephrine after 48-h starvation in humans. *The American journal of physiology*. January 1990. Accessed April 14, 2017. https://www.ncbi.nlm.nih.gov/pubmed/2405717.**

[7] **Barnosky, A. R., K. K. Hoddy, T. G. Unterman, and K. A. Varady. Intermittent fasting vs daily calorie restriction for type 2 diabetes prevention: A review of human findings. Translational Research: *The Journal of Laboratory and Clinical Medicine*. October 2014. Accessed April 14, 2017.** https://www.ncbi.nlm.nih.gov/pubmed/24993615.

[8] **Varady, K. A. Intermittent versus daily calorie restriction: Which diet regimen is more effective for weight loss? Obesity Reviews: *An Official Journal of the International Association for the Study of Obesity*. July 2011. Accessed April 14, 2017.** https://www.ncbi.nlm.nih.gov/pubmed/21410865.

[9] **Women & Diabetes. DiabetesSisters. 2012. Accessed April 15, 2017. https://diabetessisters.org/women-diabetes.**

[10] **Heart disease in women: Understand symptoms and risk factors. Mayo Clinic. June 14, 2016. Accessed April 16, 2017. http://www.mayoclinic.org/diseases-conditions/heart-disease/in-depth/heart-disease/art-20046167.**

[11] **Varady, K. A., S. Bhutani, E. C. Church, and M. C. Klempel. Short-term modified alternate-day fasting: A novel dietary strategy for weight loss and cardioprotection in obese adults. The American journal of clinical nutrition. November 2009. Accessed April 16, 2017. https://www.ncbi.nlm.nih.gov/pubmed/19793855.**

[12] **Alirezaei, Mehrdad, Christopher C. Kemball, Claudia T. Flynn, Malcolm R. Wood, J. Lindsay Whitton, and William B. Kiosses. Short-term fasting induces profound neuronal autophagy. *Autophagy*. August 16, 2010. Accessed April 16, 2017. https://www.ncbi.nlm.nih.gov/pmc/articles/PMC3106288/.**

[13] **Wolfe, D. M., J. H. Lee, A. Kumar, S. Lee, S. J. Orenstein, and R. A. Nixon. Autophagy failure in Alzheimer's disease and the role of defective lysosomal acidification. *The European Journal of Neuroscience*. June 2013. Accessed April 16, 2017. https://www.ncbi.nlm.nih.gov/pubmed/23773064.**

[14] **Siegel, I., T. L. Liu, N. Nepomuceno, and N. Gleicher. Effects of short-term dietary restriction on survival of mammary ascites tumor-bearing rats. *Cancer Investigation*. Accessed April 16, 2017. https://www.ncbi.nlm.nih.gov/pubmed/3245934.**

[15] **Lee, C., L. Raffaghello, S. Brandhorst, F. M. Safdie, G. Bianchi, A. Martin-Montalvo, V. Pistoia, M. Wei, S. Hwang, A. Merlino, L. Emionite, R. De, and V. D. Longo. Fasting cycles retard growth of tumors and sensitize a range of cancer cell types to chemotherapy. *Science Translational Medicine*. March 07, 2012. Accessed April 16, 2017. https://www.ncbi.nlm.nih.gov/pubmed/22323820.**

[16] **Hunter, G. R., N. M. Byrne, B. Sirikul, J. R. Fernández, P. A. Zuckerman, B. E. Darnell, and B. A. Gower. Resistance training conserves fat-free mass and resting energy expenditure following weight loss. *Obesity* (Silver Spring, Md.). May 2008. Accessed April 17, 2017.**

https://www.ncbi.nlm.nih.gov/pubmed/18356845.

[17] **Alwasel, S. H., Z. Abotalib, J. S. Aljarallah, C. Osmond, S. M. Alkharaz, I. M. Alhazza, G. Badr, and D. J. Barker. Changes in placental size during Ramadan. *Placenta*. July 2010. Accessed April 17, 2017. https://www.ncbi.nlm.nih.gov/pubmed/20621763.**

[18] **Soeters, Maarten R., Nicolette M. Lammers, Peter F. Dubbelhuis, Mariëtte Ackermans, Cora F. Jonkers-Schuitema, Eric Fliers, Hans P. Sauerwein, and Johannes M Aerts. Maarten R Soeters. *The American Journal of Clinical Nutrition*. November 01, 2009. Accessed April 17, 2017. http://ajcn.nutrition.org/content/90/5/1244.abstract.**

[19] **Dhurandhar, Emily J., John Dawson, Amy Alcorn, Lesli H. Larsen, Elizabeth A. Thomas, Michelle Cardel, Ashley C. Bourland, Arne Astrup, Marie-Pierre St-Onge, James O. Hill, Caroline M. Apovian, and James M. Shikany. Emily J. Dhurandhar. The effectiveness of breakfast recommendations on weight loss: A randomized controlled trial. *The American Journal of Clinical Nutrition*. Accessed April 17, 2017. http://ajcn.nutrition.org/content/early/2014/06/04/ajcn.114.089573.abstract.**

[20] **Johnstone, A. M., P. Faber, E. R. Gibney, M. Elia, G. Horgan, B. E. Golden, and R. J. Stubbs. Effect of an acute fast on energy compensation and feeding behaviour in lean men and women. *International Journal of Obesity and Related Metabolic Disorders: Journal of the International Association for the Study of Obesity*. December 2002. Accessed April 17, 2017. https://www.ncbi.nlm.nih.gov/pubmed/12461679.**

CPSIA information can be obtained
at www.ICGtesting.com
Printed in the USA
FSHW011553081218
54336FS